Calcium and Phosphorus Foods

"Deficiency or Excesses in These Minerals Cause Bone and Brain Power Loss – Don't Lose Either One"

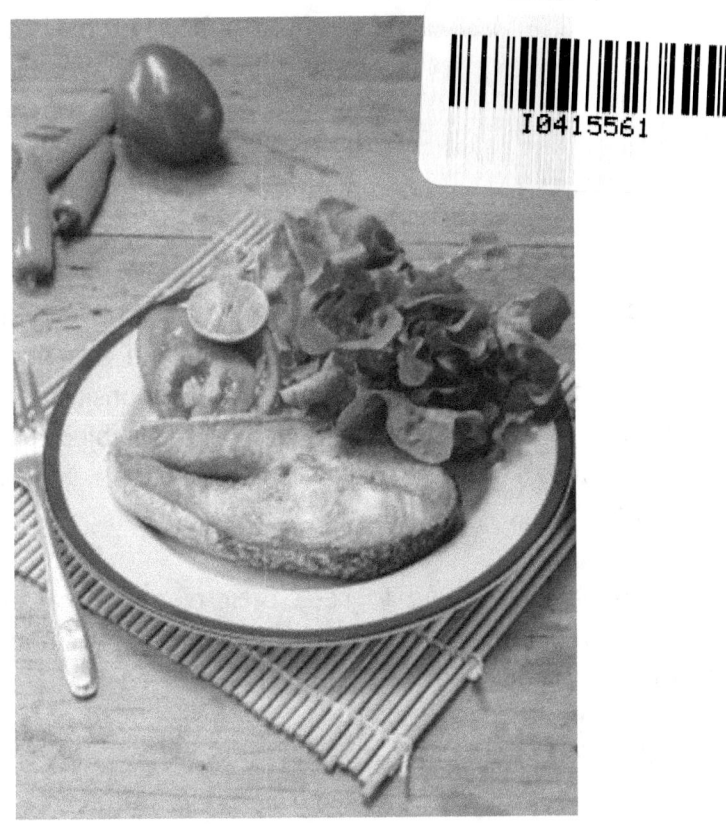

Rudy S. Silva, Natural Nutritionist

TABLE OF CONTENTS

THE MIRACLE OF CALCIUM

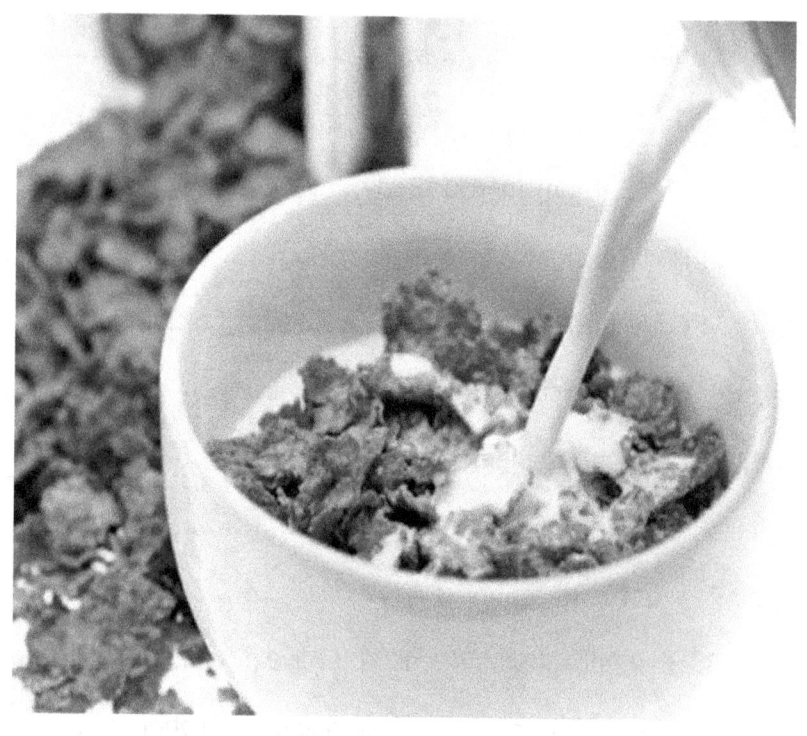

CHAPTER 1: THE CALCIUM IN YOUR BODY

Calcium occurs in the earth as limestone, calcium carbonate, as gypsum, or as apatite. It is always found combined with other elements. You will never find a pure calcium rock.

When these types of calcium compounds combine with water, they dissolve and form an alkaline solution. This is one of the reasons why you want to know as much about calcium, since it is one of the main elements that can make your body liquids alkaline. One of the most important health programs you need to pursue is to move your body from an acid condition into an alkaline condition and calcium helps you do this.

When your body is maintained consistently in an acid condition, calcium is also consistently removed from your bones, which results in porous bones, or from tissue or organs causing degradation of those areas.

Calcium is the most abundant of the minerals in your body and it makes up 1.6% of your body weight or represents 40% of all of the minerals in your body. But, 99% of the calcium you have is located in your bones. The other 1% is distributed throughout your body, and it's involved in numerous structural and biochemical processes throughout your body.

Bone Loss

Bone loss starts around middle age. For women it increases during menopause. For men, bone loss is slow but steady starting from around 30. In bone loss there are normally no symptoms. But here are a few that stand out:

- ❖ Bone deformity or rickets

- ❖ Muscle and leg cramps
- ❖ Insomnia
- ❖ Growth retardation

Unfortunately, around 40% of women who live over 75 years will experience bone loss factures. Here are some reasons for low bone mass at any age.

- ❖ Diet that lacks daily use of fruits and vegetables
- ❖ Slender body or low weight
- ❖ Premature menopause
- ❖ Anorexia nervosa
- ❖ Extreme athletic training
- ❖ Lack of exercise or a sedentary lifestyle
- ❖ Excess eating or using various types of meat or protein, phosphorus, sodium, caffeine, wheat bran, and alcohol
- ❖ Smoking
- ❖ Excess use of sodas
- ❖ Use of corticosteroid medications
- ❖ Prolong bed rest or confined to a wheel chair

It has been found that if you lack a small drop in the required level of calcium in your body this deficiency will activate aging and many degenerative diseases. Even though calcium is a large atom, it chemically moves 10,000 times faster and is 10,000 times stronger than magnesium. This gives calcium the ability to bind quickly and strongly with important biological molecules, which sustain life. This chemical flexibility gives calcium the honor of being called "the King of the Bioelements."

In this book, you will discover why it has been named King of the Bioelements. Despite there is more calcium in the body than any other mineral, with exception of oxygen, calcium is not more important than the other minerals, since all work together and are needed in your body for maintaining life.

What we can say about calcium is that it is involved in more biochemical activities in your body than any other mineral, so that it is important to supply your body with a good amount of calcium. Your body will eliminate the excess calcium from your body as its natural behavior, even when it is in a super saturated form in your body liquids.

But when there is a deficiency of other minerals in your body that must balance with calcium, like sodium, excess calcium can react un-naturally, causing calcium crystalline deposits, which lead to pain and disease.

When your body lacks calcium and has weak or porous bones, calcium will deposit calcium crystalline stones in various places in your body as it tries to build up weak bones. A misconception is that if you have calcium deposits in the joints or tissue giving you pain, that you have too much calcium.

The truth is you do not have enough calcium, so the body tries to compensate for this by calcium deposit to build your bones back up.

Calcium is found in your blood, bone structure, tissue, muscles, lymph liquid, and in every body cell in your body. It is found in the lymph liquid outside and inside your cells. In the so called **Sodium – Potassium Pump** the mineral sodium moves out of the cell and moves potassium into the cell. When the inside of the cell has mostly potassium, the electrical charge inside the cell is less than the charge outside of the cell where sodium dominates. This condition attracts calcium to carry food nutrients into the cell and to perform in the cells various biochemical and bioelectrical reactions.

Calcium ions also play a major role in nerve stimulations and transmissions, muscle contractions and movements, and organ hormone secretions and many other biological functions. It is involved with your body's enzymes to produce energy.

Calcium ionic concentrations are the most regulated mineral in your blood plasma. Its ionic form is Ca^{++} and in this form its most important function is in nerve function. For nerve function, calcium keeps your nerves receptive to sodium ions which help to transmit brain impulses and information to various parts of the body, which regulate your body's activities.

In those cultures where drinking water had a high content of calcium, it was found that people's life span was 10 years or more than in western countries.

Kidneys

Your kidneys act as filters for your blood and they remove those nutrients or chemicals that your body no longer needs from your blood and this includes calcium. Excess calcium is routed to your bladder where it is expelled in your urine. If calcium is still needed, your kidneys will pass it into your blood to be reused by your body.

Most minerals and vitamins combine and react with calcium to produce the various body structures and chemicals that make up your body.

It was thought at one time that if you produced kidney stones that you needed to take less calcium. If you tend to form kidney stones, you will have increased calcium in your urine, but this is caused by your body pulling calcium out of your bones.

Because eating excess meat cause your body to excrete calcium it is recommended, for kidney stones, to eat less meat, increase the use of fruits and vegetables, and supplement with calcium citrate, magnesium, vitamin B6 and vitamin C.

You can take calcium citrate on an empty stomach. Most other supplements, you should take with meals.

Calcium Toxicity

Usually, there is no calcium toxicity, even when you take a large dose. There is some concern that people with a tendency toward kidney stones should avoid excess calcium, but these concerns have not been proven. Kidney stones are more related to diet and those people who favor an acid diet tend to form kidney stones. In an acid diet, calcium is active and depleted as it is used up neutralizing body acids.

CHAPTER 2: HOW CALCIUM WORKS IN YOUR BODY

Here is a list of some of the important biochemical and bioelectrical functions of calcium in the body:

- ❖ Absorption of calcium
- ❖ Activity in cell function
- ❖ Maintaining an alkaline body
- ❖ Contributing to Saliva alkaline body test
- ❖ Needed Calcium foods

Adsorption of Calcium

Calcium is one of more difficult minerals to digest and to absorb through your intestinal walls. Various phosphates and other compounds (Phosphates are derived from phosphoric acid and when they combine with oxygen they become an organic phosphates, which have important biochemical activities in your body) found in red meat and sodas react with calcium to form a calcium phosphate precipitate. This prevents calcium from being absorbed and calcium is then excreted from your body.

However, when calcium comes in contact with the food substance of milk and various fruits and vegetables, it forms compounds that are easily absorbed.

For calcium to be absorbed into your body, it needs to have adequate vitamin D. Without Vitamin D, calcium cannot be absorbed into your blood stream. Vitamin D can be obtained from the sun and is critical in the amount of calcium absorption that occurs in your small intestine. This is why you need to get at least

20 minutes of sun every day. In some parts of the world less time is needed and in other parts more time is needed.

You can also get vitamin D from supplements. Some foods have it, but in very small quantities. When the sun's UV light hits your skin, fatty acids in your skin create vitamin D and **Inositol triphosphate, INSP-3**. This vitamin D finds its way into your intestinal wall where it assists calcium to move through your intestinal walls and into your blood stream.

Inositol triphosphate finds its way into everybody cell. Its function is to release calcium from storage from within your cells, when insufficient calcium is not provided by your diet and supplements, or when insufficient vitamin D causes less calcium to be absorbed in the intestinal wall.

Inositol is obtained from foods such as fruits, vegetables, grains, and from liver, kidney and heart.

When there is insufficient calcium in the cell walls, because it got used up, the parathyroid hormone stimulated by deficiency of vitamin D activates the extraction of calcium from your bones. Once the bones become weaken, your body starts extracting calcium from proteins that regulate your cell functions. This results in a variety of aliment and disease symptoms.

Once in your blood stream, calcium is deposited in bones with the help of the hormone, calcitonin, released by parathyroid gland. Also, both Calcitonin and Inositol triphosphate regulate the storage and removal of calcium with in the cells.

The parathyroid gland is regulated by the pituitary gland, which is right behind the eyes. When you wear sunglasses this blocks the full spectrum UV light that is needed to regulate the pituitary gland, so that it can produce the hormones needed to regulate calcium in your cells.

Without adequate amounts of vitamin D, calcium will not be absorbed in proper amounts into your body and will just pass right through, excreted from your body.

Parathyroid – How it regulates calcium

The parathyroid is actively involved in maintaining your calcium blood levels. These levels are maintained to a very strict range. When your blood calcium levels drop, the parathyroid releases a hormone that directs the release of calcium from your bones and into your blood stream. And at the same time, it tells your kidneys not to excrete calcium into your urine.

Now, when you have excess calcium in your blood, the amount of the parathyroid hormone secreted is decreased. This causes the kidneys to expel more calcium into your urine. As all of this is happening, the parathyroid also releases a hormone called Calcitonin, which reduces the amount of calcium that is pull out of your bones.

Activity in cell function

Calcium is active in the process involving the Sodium-Potassium Pump in that it uses this pump to enter and exit from a cell. When it enters the cell, it brings in food nutrients to feed the cells. Once it releases these nutrients, it becomes a free ion. As these calcium ions build up in the cell, the voltage across the cell membrane will again reaches 70 millivolts. This sets the stage for nutrients and toxins in the cell to be pushed out of the cell and for other nutrients to enter the cell.

Maintaining an alkaline body

The fluid outside the cells is called extracellular fluid. This fluid is maintained at a pH of 7.4 by a calcium compound called calcium mono orthophosphate. This fluid is capable of neutralizing acids that comes out of the cells or arrive there from food that you have eaten. Sodium is also in the extracellular fluid and can neutralize acids, but it is needed in large quantities to maintain the Sodium-Potassium Pump cell activity. Wherever calcium is in the tissue, joints, blood, liquid or organs, it will neutralize acids. This process reduces damage to your tissues and elevates your body pH, making it more alkaline.

When you don't have enough calcium in your body, the cells will not have enough calcium to neutralize body acids and this will cause cell deterioration and will lead to various diseases.

Keeping your body liquid alkaline or with a pH above 6.8 to 7.5 is what you should be working towards with any health program that you are working with. This can be done by using the right alkaline diet.

An alkaline diet helps you balance the level of acid and alkaline in all parts of your body. When you eat more acid foods, such as meat, butter, fats, carbohydrates, then your body needs to use up its alkaline stores to neutralize this acid, to prevent damage to your body's cells and tissue.

When you eat more alkaline foods than you need, you run the risk of not getting enough protein or carbohydrate and your pH can move above 7. 5 or 8.0 which can also lead to disease. You need a balance of certain foods to get your body pH in the range of 7.0

The saliva alkaline body test

In other kindle books, the saliva test has been discussed so that you can check its pH. This test is a strong indicator of whether your calcium ion level is sufficient. Here is a review.

When your Saliva pH is 7.0 to 7.5 it is considered alkaline and normal. When this is the case, your urine will be slightly acidic. When you lack ionic calcium, your pH will be 4.6 to 6.4 and your urine will be tend to be acidic.

Now here is important information. If you have physical ailments, your pH will be from 6.0 to 6.5. In this case, you should take around 2000 mg of calcium rather than 1000 mg. If your pH is below 6.0, mostly likely, you will have various disease symptoms. And, you should be taking around 3000 mg of calcium. Once you bring up your salivary pH, you can lower your calcium intake.

If your saliva tests show your pH to be below 6.0 then by taking more calcium supplements and by eating more fruits and vegetable during the day and especially in the evening, you can change your pH to 6.5 to 7.5

Keep in mind that the saliva test may not always be accurate, since the saliva pH can be influenced by food recently eaten. To get the most accurate reading, take the saliva test only after 2 hours of eating your last meal or snack. Also, bring saliva into your mouth 3 times and swallow, before taking the test. Take the test 3 times on 3 different days to make sure your readings are consistent.

In my kindle e-book called "Secret Diet and Nutrition Tips 1: Alkaline Body" I show you how you can change your body from 6.0 pH to 7.0 pH. In addition, in this book I show you how to do the saliva test properly so that you can get a good reading.

Simply changing your diet, taking vitamins, and mineral supplements when you eat, you can change your body's pH to the 7.0 to 7.5 level. When you do this, you will see a change in any physical aliment and disease that you might have. It will not occur instantly. You will need to keep this pH level for a few months.

Chapter 3: Body Imbalances Caused by Lack of Calcium

Calcium plays a major role in blood, cells, liver, kidney, and heart health. Calcium maintains blood pH to 7.40, solidifies bones, and helps heal scars, and fights scurvy and germs. It is present in cartilage, fluids, and tissue. It is useful for Indigestion, headaches, muscle pains, arthritis, ileitis, colitis, asthma. Lack of calcium creates problems, symptoms, and disease in the areas mentioned above.

The one thing to remember is that calcium from food sources does not contribute to arteriosclerosis, calcium deposits, increase blood pressure, and other illnesses.

Calcium is one of the main minerals that promote healing in bones, tissue, organs, brain and in all parts of the body. It is carried to various parts of the body through the blood vessels. When you lack calcium, the infected or weaken areas do not get repaired properly and disease sets in. Without the necessary calcium your body needs, blood coagulation is affected and excess bleeding can occur.

Sun Glasses

Sunlight is a necessary energy that helps to insure the absorptions of calcium. But sunlight also plays another important role in regulating calcium throughout your body.

Sunlight or full spectrum white light plays a major role in how the pituitary and pineal glands work. In the work place however, the lighting is artificial and this has a big impact on your long term health.

The use of sunglasses is quite popular and because of the many different sunglass tints that exist, people wearing them filter out the sunlight frequencies associated with that tint. Full spectrum light, like sun light, is necessary for proper function of the pituitary and pineal glands.

In the book, The Calcium Factor: The scientific Secret of Health and youth, 2000, Robert R. Barefoot & Carl J. Reich, M.D. say,

"When artificial full spectrum lighting is used, human calcium absorption increases, plants flourish and cows produce 15% more milk...Tinted glasses can eliminate a large percentage of the sun's spectrum and therefore affect you both physically and psychologically. Thus, full spectrum light plays a vital role in the maintenance of balanced hormonal system and is therefore indispensable in maintaining a balanced calcium serum."

Osteoporosis

Osteoporosis is the lack of calcium in the bone and it is estimated that over 30% of the older population will develop this condition. This is not a condition that results from old age, but a condition that comes from having an acid body for a long time.

Since the endocrine glands exert a great amount of control over calcium, the endocrine glands are put out of balance by sugar. This causes an imbalance in calcium and then shows up as cavities in your teeth.

It is the imbalance of calcium in your body that is the start of the development of chronic illnesses.

Menstrual Flow

Menstrual blood contains up to 40 times more calcium than regular blood. If you have excessive flow then you become depleted of calcium and iron. It is during this period that you should be eating kale, using liquid chlorophyll, and the many foods outlined in this book.

Without using a program that replaces your loss of calcium and iron during your periods, you open yourself to various diseases later on.

For a diet that contains plenty of iron you can check out book called, "Quick and Easy Diet Cures 4 Iron Deficiency Anemia."

Teeth health

Your teeth are made up of calcium phosphate. They are kept healthy by your blood and the nutrients that you supply them. The external part of your teeth is protected by enamel, which is an extremely strong material. But, acids that form in your mouth, when sugar is eaten, create an excess of bacteria that can penetrate that enamel.

Having dental cavities is a sign of lack of calcium. When your body needs calcium and you have not provided enough in your diet or your calcium body stores are depleted, calcium is pulled out of your teeth and bones to bring your body back into calcium balance. This weakens the teeth and bacteria can penetrate the enamel causing tooth decay.

Arteriosclerosis

Arteriosclerosis is not caused by an excess of calcium. It is caused by the lack of sodium and chlorine salts. Calcium needs these salts to be properly used and to stay in solution and not precipitate out onto artery walls. It is needed so that artery walls don't become inflamed by acid damage and consequently need repair through plaque buildup.

Arteriosclerosis occurs when plaque builds up along the artery walls, which takes place over years. Eventually this plaque will narrow the arteries and cause reduced blood flow or blood flow blockage. Reduced blood flow will result in many different illnesses because cells will not be getting the proper oxygen and nutrition. Blockage will result in heart attacks.

Plaque is made up of phospholipids, collagen, triglycerides, fibrin mucopolysaccharides, cholesterol, heavy metals, proteins, muscle tissue, and debris, which are all bonded by calcium.

Plaque only occurs in arteries that deliver blood from the heart to your body and not in the veins that return blood to the heart. Cholesterol is not the cause of plaque, but even if it was it can be controlled by diet and not drugs. Eighty percent of the cholesterol in your body is created in the body and 20% of it comes from your diet. Your body uses cholesterol in every cell, in hormones, in nerve impulses, in the brain, and in the creation of vitamin D on your skin.

It is the cellular breakdown along the artery walls caused by acidity surrounding the wall tissue or free radical damage that prompts repair of that area and that is when plaque starts to build up on the wall.

Heart Disease

Calcium is central to good heart function. Since calcium ions are linked to proper cell function, any deterioration you have in your cell do to the lack of calcium will affect the cell structure of heart cells and to the cells of the arteries. This deterioration will lead to heart diseases.

In addition the ability of the heart to contract and expand is due to the ionization of calcium, Ca^{++}.

Effects of Excess Calcium

When your body has an excess of calcium, you will see external and internal boney growths. These growths can occur in any part of your body such as joints, tissue, organs, or muscle. The growths may appear as kidney stones or other precipitates that occur on your heels, shoulder joints, knee joints, or toe bones.

When you have excess calcium, you need to eat more fruits and vegetables to get the natural absorbable vitamins and minerals, especially sodium. Sodium and calcium must always be in balance, lack of one or the other leads to a chemical imbalance, which results in various illnesses or diseases.

Illness or Conditions Due To Lack of Calcium

Here some of the symptoms or conditions that occur when you lack calcium:

- ❖ tumors
- ❖ sores, abscesses, inflammations
- ❖ discharges
- ❖ deformed fingers, bones, hips cranial bones
- ❖ tooth decay
- ❖ undersized organs
- ❖ blood deficiencies
- ❖ back pain
- ❖ vomiting
- ❖ tuberculosis
- ❖ excess bleeding
- ❖ excess mucus discharge
- ❖ poor scar healing
- ❖ craving for salt
- ❖ bone softening
- ❖ swelling knuckles
- ❖ bronchial congestion
- ❖ wrinkled skin
- ❖ cystic goiter
- ❖ cyst formation
- ❖ nervous problems

There are so many illness and poor body conditions that occur when you lack calcium. You may have a few of these, but if they are consistent and they remain with you for a while, consider increasing your calcium intake.

Nervous Problems

Anxiety is supposed to help you when you are involved in stressful or life threating situation. Under these conditions your metabolism increases, muscles tighten, and you get a shot of adrenaline. When anxiety happens, you use up many minerals, including calcium. Under stressful conditions that last more than a day, it is wise to take a calcium supplement.

Back pain

Back pain is one of those conditions that when it occurs it can disable you and cause you to take a quick trip to emergency. When back pain is caused by strained muscles, stress, bad posture, in activity, or lack of exercise, one of the supplements recommend is calcium with magnesium. These minerals reduce muscle spasms, muscle tightness, and nerve irritation.

Taking a supplement that contains calcium, magnesium, and vitamin D daily, will help you to alleviate the long list of body conditions or illnesses. Just remember that calcium is a relaxer and nerve reliever.

CHAPTER 4: EATING CALCIUM FOODS

Even though you eat calcium foods, only around 25% of the calcium in this food will be absorbed by your body. But as a child or if you are pregnant, you may absorb up to 60%.

When cooking fruits or vegetables, you should use lower temperatures, when possible. When produce is heated to above 150 Fahrenheit at least 33% of the available calcium is lost.

Calcium and Milk

All milk that is pasteurized at high temperature is a low source of calcium. There is some milk that is pasteurized at 145 degrees Fahrenheit that are better sources of calcium. All milk that has been pasteurized or homogenized is acidic. The best milk source for calcium is raw goat milk and since it has not been heated it is alkaline in nature.

Despite the insistence from The Dairy Council that,

"Milk has been part of the diet for thousands of years. Despite the fact that milk is one of the most nutritionally complete foods available, there are many myths relating its consumption that blame milk and dairy foods for a variety of ailments. Many of these myths have been part of the folklore for centuries and are not founded on science."

There is tremendous amount of scientific papers and finding that milk should not be included in your diet, because of the illnesses it contributes too. But then again there are studies that show there is a decrease in heart and cancer in people that drink milk.
An article, In 1992 The New England Journal of Medicine pointed out that, "Consumption of cow's milk has been associated with insulin dependent diabetes..."

But this is also evidence that some milk should be drunk and that there are other sources of dairy products that can provide plenty of calcium for your diet, such as yogurt or cottage cheese.

Because of the tremendous activity of calcium in the body in relation to cell nutrition and it alkalizing effect, it is best to eat plenty of those vegetables and fruits that are high in calcium.

In his book, **Prescription for Natural Cures**, 2004, by James F. Balch, M.D. he says,

"It may surprise you to learn that countries where people drink the most milk are also those with the highest rates of osteoporosis. This may be due to the fact that lactose intolerance and casein allergy are very common and lead to mal-absorption. Also, calcium from cow's milk is not well absorbed, at a rate of 25 percent. Milk products lead to other health problems as well, so don't rely on them as source calcium. Unsweetened, cultured yogurt is an exception."

One way to eat your unsweetened yogurt is to add it to a blender and then add fruits like strawberries, pineapple, mango, bananas, and so on. To get additional sweetness, you can add some raw honey, since honey helps you to absorb calcium.

The British Medical Research Council made a 10 year study of 5000 men aged 45 to 59. In this study they found, "only 1 percent of those who regularly drank more than one-half liter of milk a day suffered heart attacks ... against 10 per cent of those who drank no milk at all."

In this study, researchers also found there was no difference whether they drank pure milk or skimmed, the benefits were still there.

There is still a lot of controversy about drinking milk for calcium. If you feel good drinking milk, then you should drink it. If you develop mucus or other symptoms, when you drink milk, then you should consider getting your calcium from other sources.

Where you can get calcium

One of the highest sources of calcium comes from **barley, green kale,** and **turnip greens**. You can get good calcium from cereals and grains.

Here is a list of foods highest in calcium:

- Seaweed – dulse, kelp, Irish moss, wakame, nori, sombu, agar
- Sardines with bones
- Tempeh, tofu
- Avocados, figs, prunes
- All dark greens, collard greens, spinach, kale,
- Unprocessed seeds and nuts – sesame seeds, grains, and nuts, almonds, walnuts
- Bone broth
- Cows, skimmed milk, cheese, cottage cheese, goat milk, yogurt
- Rice milk-calcium enriched
- Cabbage, cauliflower, celery, lemons, rhubarb
- Egg yolk, gelatin foods
- Fish, meat near the bone
- Whole wheat bread
- Beans, brown rice, lentils, millet, oats,
- Broccoli, Brussels sprouts, cauliflower
- Onions, parsnips, watercress
- Raw butter, gelatin, blackstrap molasses
- Coconut, raw cream, egg yolk
- Fish, meat near the bone, bone broth
- Natural cane sugar

The amount of calcium in certain foods

½ cup of wakame – sea vegetable gives 1700 mg

¼ cup of agar – sea vegetable gives 1000 mg

½ cup of nori – sea vegetable gives 600 mg

¼ cup of kombu – sea vegetable gives 500 mg

1 cup of tempeh gives 340 mg

8 oz. of calcium enriched rice milk give 300 mg

1 cup of almonds gives 300 mg

8 oz. of skim milk gives 302 mg

8 oz. of low fat yogurt gives 300 mg

1 oz. of Swiss cheese gives 272 mg

10 figs give 269 mg

½ cup of tofu gives 258 mg

½ cup of sesame seeds gives 250 mg

1 oz. of mozzarella cheese gives 183 mg

½ cup of boiled collards gives 179 mg

1 tablespoon of blackstrap molasses gives 172 mg

1 cup cottage cheese gives 126 mg

2 sardines in oil give 92 mg

¼ cup of walnuts gives 70 mg

1 cup of black beans or lentils gives 55 mg

½ cup of boiled mustard greens gives 52 mg

½ cup of boiled broccoli gives 36 mg

Dark Greens

The dark greens can be boiled instead of steamed and their taste is improved. Boiling them also does not cause them to reduce their nutritional value, since they has such high nutrition to begin with.

Meat

Limit the amount of meat you eat. Meat has 30 times more phosphorous than calcium. And, in the digestive tract, this phosphorous will cause the calcium to precipitate to form apatite, which is a form of a phosphorous calcium mineral crystal. It is apatite that is the substance that forms your bones. The result is that this calcium is not available to you and is excreted from your body.

Sugar

It has been found that there is 40% less calcium in white sugar as compared to raw sugar. Blackstrap molasses has 258 times more calcium as white sugar. Calcium and sugar attract each other. The more sugar you eat the more calcium is precipitated. The less body calcium you have the more tooth decay you will have.

Salt

Using excess salt in your food has been associated with bone loss. If you eat salt with your food, salt competes with calcium to get absorbed. The more salt is absorbed the less calcium is.

Try using culinary herbs and chili sauces to flavor your food. If you like salty food, you could use them as a snack and not with your regular meals.

Nightshades

Foods like tomatoes, potatoes, eggplant, peppers and tobacco, which are considered nightshade foods.

In her book, Food and Healing, 1986, Annemarie Colbin points out that,

"In my own experience and that of some of my students, consuming nightshades on a dairy-free diet has resulted in a loss of calcium, evidenced by brittle nails, painful gums, and dental caries. Eliminating the nightshades, rather than increasing the dairy, solved the problem"

There are some foods that promote the excretion of calcium. We have indicated that eating excess meat can trap calcium and eliminate it from your body.

Foods high in oxalic acid also promote the removal of calcium from your body – spinach, cranberries, and rhubarb.

Wheat bran also limits the amount of calcium you absorb because to the phytic acid in its fiber. The phytic acid in wheat fiber has the ability to combine with calcium and limit its absorption in your body.

Other things that limit your calcium absorption are eating too many foods that contain phosphorus, drinking tea which contains tannins, lack of vitamin D, and having diarrhea.

Pumpkin Seeds

Shelled pumpkin seeds are a high source of zinc, magnesium, iron phosphorus, and calcium. You can eat a hand full every day.

CHAPTER 5: CALCIUM SUPPLEMENTS

Taking calcium supplements is a great idea, since you are probably not getting all of the calcium you need in your diet.

However, since calcium tends to interfere with the absorption of other minerals, it is best to also take a multivitamin that provides those other minerals.

What type of calcium supplements should you take? A good supplement is one that contains:

- ❖ Calcium 1000 – 1500 mg
- ❖ Magnesium 400 – 600 mg
- ❖ Vitamin D in Cholecalciferol form, called D3

So what are your daily requirements for calcium? Daily requirements for calcium are between 1000 to 1500mg. The type of supplement and the amount you take depends on your ability to absorb calcium. This is difficult to determine, so it is best to take the high end of calcium – 1500 mg.

Here are some minimum calcium supplementation requirements. Keep in mind that if you can get this amount in your food then you don't need to take calcium supplements.

Infants 7-12 months   270 mg

Children 4-8 years   800mg

Males 31-50   1000mg

Females 31-50   1000mg

Pregnant and lactating 1000mg

One of the best calcium supplements to use is Brazil Live Coral. It contains calcium, vitamin D, magnesium, and all of the trace minerals. It is in powder form so it is more absorbable. It contains the vitamin D you need to absorb the calcium. But you also need to spend at least 20 to 30 minutes in the sun to get the natural vitamin D. It does not have to be in the direct sunlight, but it is better, if you can do it. Look on the internet for:

Brazil Live Coral

Also look for **Okinawa coral calcium** which is another good product.

Another excellent calcium supplement is called, **3-Way Calcium Complex™.** Look for this on the internet. It uses three different forms of calcium and includes other nutrients that help you absorb more of this calcium.

Calcium absorption

For calcium to be absorbed in the body, it is crucial to have adequate vitamin D in your body. Without Vitamin D, calcium cannot be absorbed into your body. Vitamin D can be obtained from the sun and from supplements. Be aware that wearing sunglasses can affect your health by not keeping your pituitary gland healthy.

It's the pituitary gland that tells the parathyroid to release hormones that help to regulate and absorb calcium. In addition to eating calcium foods, take Brazil Live Coral Calcium and also add vitamin D as a supplement to your diet, especially if you don't go out into sun every day.

Vitamin C

It is believed that by taking vitamin C with Calcium, you increase the absorption of calcium. A form of calcium that is already combined with vitamin C is called Calcium Ascorbate. This type of calcium is easily transported across the intestinal walls.

Chelated calcium

It is best to use calcium supplements in chelated form. What this means is that calcium is tied to an amino acid and this makes it easier for calcium to pass through your intestinal walls. Chelated calcium is more easily absorbed than calcium that is not chelated. Here are some of the types of calcium amino acid chelates you should look for and buy.

Calcium Alpha Keto Glucarate

Calcium ascorbate – a form of calcium that is tied to vitamin C

Calcium Lactate

Calcium Arginate

Calcium hydroxyapatite – the type of calcium found in your bones

Calcium Glycinate

Calcium Amino Acid Chelate

Calcium Caprylate

Calcium Malate

Calcium Gluconate

Calcium L-Aspartate

Calcium Lactate Gluconate

Calcium Lysinate

Calcium Orotate

Calcium Succinate

Tri calcium phosphate – the type of calcium in your bones

All of these amino acids tied to calcium can also be attached to the other minerals like magnesium and potassium. So you can find magnesium arginate or magnesium alginate or magnesium aspartate.

Honey

It has been found by the United States Department of Agriculture nutritionist Richard J. Wood that the glucose in honey can increase your absorption of calcium by up to 25%. It can also increase the absorption of zinc and magnesium.

Types of Calcium to avoid

Calcium Dolomite

Avoid using dolomite as a source of calcium, since it may not be absorbed properly by your body. Dolomite is a form of calcium carbonate and magnesium.

Calcium carbonate

Calcium carbonate is hard to absorb when the pH in your stomach is not at the proper level. If you low levels of stomach acid you will not be able to absorb this type of calcium.

Magnesium

Magnesium is usually found in calcium supplements because it is required for proper calcium metabolism. Magnesium has a role in the formation of bones. It has been found that when there is a decrease in blood magnesium that there is also a drop in blood calcium. The lack of magnesium in your body can increase the risk of osteoporosis.

Magnesium's absorption is enhanced by vitamin D just like calcium is. Magnesium is active in making sure that cells function properly by moving sodium and potassium in and out of the cells. Magnesium, just like calcium, is important for nerve and heart function. Many of the foods that are high in calcium are also high in magnesium.

CHAPTER 6: HOW CALCIUM BURNS ACID

In this chapter, you will discover how you can make your body more alkaline. Calcium in addition to other minerals is one of the main minerals that can help you do this. Keeping your body alkaline is one of the best ways to keep your body calcium levels in balance.

Minerals

Moving your body more toward alkalinity is what will give you the best curative effects of fruits. An alkaline body prevents your body from becoming ill and forming deadly diseases, like all kinds of joint problems, organ degradation, body pain, or even cancer. If you are already sick, then all of the chemicals inside fruits will help to revive you to better health. This is provided that your tissue damage has not gone beyond repair.

The minerals most important in changing and maintaining your body in an alkaline condition are sodium, potassium, chloride, calcium, phosphorus, magnesium, and sulfur.

Now, how your body can become alkaline might become a little confusing at first because of the terms used, but let's break this down into small parts. This process has been discussed in previous chapters, but this explanation gives more details. First we are going to be defining some terms so we can then start talking the same language.

Acid Binding

There are certain minerals that are called acid binding. And these are minerals, as mentioned earlier, are the most important ones in fruits, Sodium, potassium, chloride, calcium, phosphorus, magnesium, because they are acid binding.

What acid binding means is when you eat fruits with these minerals, your cells, after metabolism, create an alkaline ash. This ash will seek out acids in your body and bind with them to neutralize them.

Alkaline Ash

Now, that this alkaline forming ash has tied up an acid it is carried to the kidney where it is expelled as urine.

Different reactions can occur when an acid binding mineral, like say sodium, encounters an acid. Of course acids in the body are toxic, so the body has the priority of getting rid of them fast, since they can damage tissue and cause pain and disease.

Here is another path way of the acid binding mineral process when it combines with an acid.

The Acid Binding Mineral Process

When you eat acid binding food, the blood carries it to the cells where it is oxidized, digested, or metabolized. The result of this digestion is a carbonic acid salt of alkaline minerals, which reacts with body acids and binds with them. In this process, a weak carbonic acid is created. Now, this weak carbonic acid is taken by the blood into the lungs where it is released as carbon dioxide and water.

If not all the acid toxins are captured by acid binding matter, the remaining acids can be neutralized by body stores of alkaline minerals. If you don't have a good store of alkaline minerals, then these acids will remain in your body creating pain and disease.

But if you do have a good store of alkaline minerals, then these minerals will find these acids, capture them and bind with them. Then these acids are routed out through your urine or colon and out of your body.

So you can see the importance of getting a lot of alkaline minerals into your body. Without them, acids which do not get bonded to alkaline minerals would move back into body tissue and continue their body damage.

Alkaline Binding

Now, there are also minerals that become alkaline binding and these minerals are sulphur, chlorine, iodine, phosphorous, bromine, fluorine, copper, and silicon.

It is these minerals that when digested by a cell will produce an acid salt that will bind with alkaline minerals. These minerals will be excreted through your urine. When alkaline minerals are bonded to an acid salt, the alkaline mineral is removed from your body and your body becomes more acidic, the condition you are trying to avoid.

Although you need to eat both foods that are acid binding or alkaline binding, you want to eat more of the acid binding foods.

Keeping Healthy

One of the most important parts of health is keeping the lymph liquid around your cells clean and free of toxins. To do this you need provide alkaline minerals to occupy the lymph liquid and you need to remove the acids that accumulate in that liquid and in all parts of your body tissue. You can do this by detoxifying your body and providing alkaline minerals for your lymph liquid.

Body Detoxification

The highest priority of the body is to detoxify itself. One of the best way to help your body detoxify is to provide minerals that bind with acids that are in the cells, tissues, organs, and muscles. What these alkaline acid binding minerals do is to pull out the toxins that are dispersed throughout your body.

With the help of the liver which detoxifies the blood, the kidney that removes impurities from the blood and the lungs which removes the CO_2 which results from alkaline acid binding, your body is constantly detoxifying itself. But when it is over loaded with acid toxins from your lifestyle, a complete detox of your body becomes impossible.

Where do Acid Toxins Come From

So why is the body overloaded with toxins? Why can't the liver take care of these toxins? The liver has the function to remove acid wastes from natural food that is created by food digestion and cell metabolism. When it encounters acid wastes such as food enhancers, dyes, preservatives, pesticides, and the variety of additives, the liver does not always know how to break them down to make them harmless.

But your body does not give up so easily when it knows that the liver was not able to disintegrate food additives. What it does is it instructs calcium to bind with these toxic acids and to take them far away from the blood stream. The result is that calcium binding with acid forms a deposit and this deposit can be placed in your teeth, your joints, and as bone spurs, which grow in your feet or shoulders, vertebra, or muscle tissue. These calcium deposits are very painful, and if you have ever experience them, you know how much.

Now, we have talked about acid toxins in the body that are brought in through food and the environment. But there is another factor that creates acid in the body and that is emotions that are occur through life stresses, like work pressures, divorce, friendship problems, martial issues, and other similar problems. These emotional problems create acidic molecules that embed themselves into your tissues just like food acids.

Body Organs

All body organs function to rid the body of acid waste or toxins. Lack of alkaline binding food causes deterioration of the function of these organs. Each organ has a specific function in the elimination and neutralization of acid wastes and it does this in conjunction with alkaline acid binding minerals.

Here is the list of the fruits that have the highest alkaline minerals and the ones that you should be eating. The percentage number next to them indicates the strength of the alkaline mineral and the closer to 100% the more effective it is as an acid binding fruit. However you should be eating all of these fruit not just the ones at the top of the list.

The percentage assigned to these fruits is based on fresh fruits that are organic and that they are not cooked, canned or mixed with sugar. If they are cook or otherwise processed in some fashion, this will reduce their effectiveness as an acid binding. However, they will still be effective in acid binding.

Acid Binding Fruits With Alkaline Minerals

In the list below are fruits with alkaline minerals that create an acid binding salt your body uses to neutralize acid wastes. Fruits above 50% in value are more acid binding, which means they will more trap acid wastes.

Here is the list of fruits to eat in the order of priority.

1. **Fruits at 100% Acid Binding – Best fruits To Eat**
    Lemons, melons – any type, watermelon

2. **Fruits at 93% Acid Binding – Great fruits To Eat**
    Cantaloupes, dried dates, dried figs, limes, mango, papaya

3. **Fruits at 87% Acid Binding – Still Great Fruits To Eat**
    Kiwis, passion fruit, pineapples, raisins, umeboshi plums

4. **Fruits at 80% Acid Binding – Eat These Fruits**
    Apricots, avocados, bananas, fresh dates, fresh figs, currants, gooseberries grapes, grapefruits guavas, kumquats, nectarines, pears, persimmons, quince

5. **Fruits at 73% Acid Binding – Still Fruits To Eat**
    Apples, organs, peaches, pomegranate, raspberries, sour grapes, strawberries

6. **Fruits at 67 Acid Binding** – Still Neutralizes Acids
   Cherries

Fruits to Concentrate On

These are the fruits you should concentrate on eating. Also eat them every day, if possible, fresh lemon juice in the morning, watermelon during the day.

You can see which fruits give you the best acid binding effects and eating them 80% of your overall food intake will convert your body over to an Alkaline body.

CHAPTER 7: WHAT IS PHOSPHORUS ALL ABOUT?

If you want to have a top thinking brain, you will want to know the information in this book. What you need to know is that you don't want to be caught with a deficiency in phosphorus or an excess. You need to strive to keep a good balance of phosphorus, because without a balance, many body functions are affected and the proper level of other minerals is disrupted.

Phosphorus is the second highest mineral you have in your body. Eight five percent of it is found in your bones and teeth. The other 15% is found in your RNA, DNA and other places in your body.

Phosphorus is part of the seven alkaline producing macrominerals – calcium, sodium, potassium, magnesium, chlorine, and sulfur. There are also 50 minerals called trace minerals. Even though some of the trace minerals occur in micro amounts in our body, they have an important function in keeping you healthy.

When you find that you are deficient in a mineral, you can eat more foods that contain that mineral or you can supplement with that mineral. However, it not a good idea just to take a single mineral supplement or vitamin, since minerals and vitamins work together in a synergistic manner. Vitamins and minerals work as catalysts promoting the absorption and assimilation of other vitamins and minerals.

If you want to correct a mineral deficiency, then you need to take a supplement of that mineral with other minerals to clear that deficiency.

One of the best ways to take minerals and vitamins is to take them with food. In this fashion, the supplement you are taking can get the other vitamins or minerals it needs to be processed through your body properly. Of course, the main way to get your phosphorus or other minerals is through eating organic fruits and vegetables.

Taking Phosphorus

When you take a phosphorus supplement, you also need to take calcium, iron, manganese, sodium and B6. So how do you do that? You need to take phosphorus or any mineral supplement with food.

It is important that all minerals used by your body be in balance. When you have too much or too little of any mineral, your health will be affected. It is the function of your elimination channels to get rid of the excess minerals and it is your job to take care of mineral deficiencies.

What Does Phosphorus Do In Your Body?

Here is what phosphorus does in your body. In your blood, it is needed for blood clotting. It is used to form teeth and bone. In your heart it is needed for contractions and to keep your heart beating normal. Your cells use it for cell growth and creating energy. It is needed for kidney function. Phosphorus helps your body to use vitamins and converts food to energy.

Your Brain On Phosphorus

All parts of your brain depend on phosphorus to function properly – nerve networks, nervous system, and ganglia. High levels of thinking depend on phosphorus – psychic perceptions, idealistic thinking, and humanitarianism. With sulphur and omega fats, phosphorus vitalizes and regenerates your brain and nerves.

Without phosphorus you could not read, reason, create, visualize, study, memorize, or comprehend. Is this a mineral you want to be caught short on? Of course not and that is why in the following chapters, you will discover how you can increase your level of blood phosphorous and at the same improve you overall level of thinking and logic.

CHAPTER 8: HOW PHOSPHORUS KEEPS YOU ALIVE

"Phosphorous is an essential brain nutrient"

Phosphorous is the major negative charged ion that exists throughout your body. Around 86% of it is found in your bones and teeth, 13% is in your soft tissue, and around 1% exists in the liquid outside of your cells, extracellular fluid. Outside the body, it is a highly toxic, nonmetallic, yellowish white element, which is insoluble in water, does not conduct electricity and has a low melting point of 110 deg F.

In your body phosphorous exist mostly as a phosphate ion in the following inorganic combination:

Calcium phosphate
Sodium phosphate
Magnesium phosphate
Iron phosphate
Potassium phosphate

In this book, when we use the word phosphorus, it refers to one of the phosphate ions listed above.

Your body contains around two pounds of phosphorus. Aside from working with calcium to create bone structures, phosphorus also supports reactions with B vitamins, nerve and muscle movement, cell division, transmitting hereditary traits, and digestion of food products at the cell level.

Here are the major functions of phosphorous:

Makes up part of your cell membrane as phospholipids
Holds DNA together
Coats nerves of the brain
Works in muscle activity
Assists in brain and neurologic functions
Acts as a tonic for brain and nerves
Maintains higher intelligence and promotes idealistic ideas
Assists carbohydrate, protein, and fat metabolism
Assists in the production of cell energy, ATP
Helps create red blood cells
Assists in buffering acids and bases
Works in white blood cell phagocytosis and platelet functions
Combines with calcium to form and repair bone matrix
Improves the reproduction systems
Helps to maintain the body's pH levels
Forms new tissue and hair.

Because phosphorus is heavily involved in building bones, it's important that children get the required amount.

Phosphorus and Your Brain

One of the greatest functions of phosphorus is to help you maintain a high level of thinking. Phosphorous is burned up during heavy mental activity, such as concentration, hard studying, long and intense mental work, excess fears, drudgery, excess drive to make money or succeed, or to be better than the next person.

When you use up phosphorus, the phosphate wastes must be eliminated by the liver. It has been found that if you do a lot of mental activity, you will have more phosphorus in your urine than normal. With this type of loss, you need to make sure you are getting plenty of phosphorus in your diet.

If you are a student at any level, you need phosphorus every day. If you don't get phosphorus, your brain softens, wilts, and decays. Neuralgia develops and intelligence disappears.

To become more intelligent and have higher levels of thinking you need to have the highest levels of phosphorus in your body, without it affecting the balance of other minerals.

What is Lecithin?

Phosphorus is needed to produce lecithin, which is a complex fatty nutrient that you must have in your body. Without lecithin, you will become impotent, will get neuratrophia, will experience brain decomposition, have feeblemindedness, and have low nerve vitality. Taking lecithin daily in your diet helps to lessen the use of phosphorus and make it available for brain nutrition.

There are two types of phosphorous, one for the high level thinking your brain does and the other for building bones.

Types of Phosphorus Food

They type of food that you need for bones come from vegetables and fruits and what you need for the brain and nervous system must come from eggs, meat, fish, chicken, turkey, birds, and dairy. It is animal products that contain lecithin, which is a fat that carry phosphorus and nutrients the brain needs. Phosphorus from meat carries a high vibrational frequency that is needed by your brain.

Vegetable do not have lecithin and carry a low amount of phosphorous, which is not enough for the body's needs.

Since the brain works at a fast speed, it uses a phosphorous that is capable of working at the speed of light. This is why brain phosphorous must come from animal meat, which vibrates at a higher level than vegetable phosphorous.

The word Lecithin comes from Greek, which means egg yolk. It is a fatty compound that is needed throughout your body. It is contained in cell membrane, nerve tissue, brain, bile, semen, white and red blood corpuscles, lymph and serous fluids, and blood. Lecithin cannot be produced by your body, so you need to provide it through your food or by supplementation.

The phosphorescent glow many insects, fish, and other animals emit comes from the large quantities of phosphorous they have. The energy the phosphorous molecule captures from outside itself allows it to release light or photons and in doing so provide the energy for the brain to do its work at the speed of light. As light is released in your brain, your head would appear to glow, if you were sensitive enough to see the millions of small emissions of light going on all of the time.

Without phosphorous, we could not reason or comprehend. As you think and as information is being sent to different parts of your body, phosphorous is being used by your brain.

Research has shown that after excessive mental exertion phosphates are broken down, processed by the liver and kidney and show up as excess phosphorous in the urine.

Body Regulation of Phosphorous

The amount of phosphorous that your body maintains is based on:

What you eat

Your hormonal regulation

What your kidney excretes through urine

Cell regulation

After your Jejunum, a part of your small intestine, absorbs phosphorous and circulates it in your blood, your kidneys eliminate the un-needed phosphorus. Your gastrointestinal tract will also excrete a small amount of phosphorus. Your gastrointestinal tract starts at your mouth and ends at your anus. So if you increase the amount of phosphorous foods or supplements you eat, your kidney adjusts the amount of phosphorous your body keeps. But, if you lack phosphorous, your kidneys – nephrons - reabsorb phosphorous from the proximal tubules in an effort to bring phosphorous levels back to normal.

Nephron means kidney and is the basic structural and functional section of the kidney. Its major function is to regulate the amount of water and various minerals your body needs by filtering your blood and excreting what your body does not need.

A nephron cleans your blood by eliminating blood waste and contaminates. It regulates blood volume, pressure, electrolytes, metabolites, and pH. The nephron is regulated by the endocrine system hormones – parathyroid hormone, antidiuretic hormone, and aldosterone.

The parathyroid gland also controls the level of phosphorous in your body. It does this by monitoring the calcium level by controlling the parathyroid hormone, PTH, since calcium and phosphorous must exist in your body in a certain ratio. When calcium levels drop, phosphorous levels must increase. PTH is released by the parathyroid causing an increase in calcium and phosphorous, which is obtained from your bones. Suppressing the PTH activity causes deposition of calcium and phosphorous back into the bones.

Phosphorous levels are also increased by calcitriol that is found in your intestinal walls, which helps phosphorous to easily pass through the intestines. Calcitriol is activated vitamin D, which are really a hormone and not a vitamin. The vitamin D that is created on the skin goes through several chemical changes to become calcitriol or activated vitamin D. It is this form of vitamin D that is attracted to the intestinal walls where it assists calcium and phosphorous to quickly and easily pass into your blood stream.

If two much phosphorous accumulates in the lymph and blood, the kidney, acted upon by the PTH, increases the excretion of phosphorous through the urine. Low levels of PTH allow the kidney to reabsorb phosphorous from the blood instead of excreting it.

Phosphorous levels can also be depleted or changed by moving in and out of cells. In the case of alkalosis, - body liquids and blood exceed a pH of 7.4 alkalinity - phosphorous is used to drop down the pH in cells and in the blood. Also when insulin moves into the cells to carry in glucose, it also drags in phosphorous causing the cell extracellular fluid to become more alkaline. So the amount of insulin active in cell activity also affects the levels of phosphorous.

Hypo phosphatemia (Insufficient Phosphorus)

Hypophosphatemia happens when the serum phosphorus level falls below 1.8mEq/L. Serum phosphorus refers to the amount of this element in your blood plasma, which is that part of the blood that is clear, sticky and contains no blood cells, platelets, or fibrinogen. If your serum phosphorus level falls below 0.8 mEq/L, your body would not have the energy to provide organ function.

How do you get to the point where you lack phosphorous in your body? There are at least four ways.

Movement of phosphorous in cell structure
Decrease of phosphorous adsorption
Decrease kidney reabsorption
Lack of phosphorus from diet

Movement of phosphorous in cell structure

The movement of phosphorous from extracellular liquid into intracellular liquid occurs under many conditions. This happens during hyperventilation, alcohol withdrawal, heat stroke, pain, anxiety, diabetic ketoacidosis, and acute slicylate poisoning. When you have excess glucose in your blood, the pancreas releases insulin to remove this excess and move it into your cells. In this process, insulin moves glucose into your cells but it also moves phosphorous with it.

When phosphorous is moved into your cells, the phosphorous levels outside the cells fall and phosphorous from the blood is released to rebalance this loss. But then blood phosphorous levels drop and need to be replaced from your bones, food, or wherever it can be found in your body.

Decrease of phosphorous adsorption

When you have poor adsorption or are starved, your body phosphorous levels will drop. When you use antacids or sucralfate – a drug for ulcers - they bind with phosphorous and decrease it below normal levels. Use of laxative can also cause excess phosphorous to be excreted in feces. Lack of vitamin D is another cause of phosphorous not being absorbed. Vitamin D in the intestine is necessary to pull phosphorous through the intestinal walls.

The following drugs can bind with phosphorous and decrease it movement into your body:

Acetazolamide
Thiazide diuretics
Chlorothiazide
Hydrochlorothiazide
Loop diuretics
Bumetanide
Furosemide
Antacids
Aluminum carbonate
Aluminum hydroxide
Calcium carbonate
Magnesium oxide
Insulin
Laxatives

Decrease kidney reabsorption

Use of diuretics is the most common cause of phosphorous loss through the kidneys. People with diabetic ketoacidosis and poor control of blood glucose levels have increase urine output, causing loss of phosphorous. Burn victims also exhibit a high loss of phosphorous. This may be a result of excess urination.

Lack of phosphorus from diet

A poor diet can contribute to low levels of phosphorus in your blood. This can be easily corrected by knowing what foods are highest in phosphorus and concentrating on these foods for a certain time period.

CHAPTER 9: SICKNESSES RELATED TO INSUFFICIENT PHOSPHORUS

When you lack phosphorus, it's called hypophosphatemia and typically it's a result from a poor diet or from a catabolic state where you exercise too much or when you fast or go without food for a long time. If you drink too much alcohol, you probably are low in phosphorus.

Here are some more reasons why you might low in phosphorus.

Intestinal malabsorption
Chronic diarrhea
Hypomagnesemia
Deficient in vitamin D – necessary for phosphorus absorption
Chronic use of antacids
Kidney tubular defects
Diabetic acidosis
Injured cells releasing phosphorus

Here are a few symptoms of **Hypophosphatemia**:

If you are suffering from lack of phosphorous, your body will exhibit a variety of symptoms. You will have:

anorexia
Low tissue oxygenation
Constant faintness
Lack of appetite or extreme hunger
Weak sexual system
Nerve pain

Difficulty reasoning with headaches
A weak nervous system
A Mental states going from apprehension to laughter
Mood changes from happiness to sadness
Increased Emotional needs: love, affection, acceptance
A need for sympathy, and acknowledgment
Bone deformations
Poor blood formation
Muscle weakness
Tremors
Impaired red blood cell functions

Personality changes occur rapidly from calmness to hysteria, when you lack phosphorus and your brain does not function well and confusion dominates. Night time brings fear and depression. Any noises disturb you. You become disgusted with yourself and those around you. Your choice of foods changes and you dislike foods you once liked. You develop a lack of confidence.

Bone deformations

If you lack phosphorus, you will not be able to properly grow bones. It is associated with rickets in children and osetomalacia, softening of bones, in adults.

Blood

Phosphorus plays a role in the formation of red, white blood cells, and platelets. Lack of phosphorus affects the amount of red blood cells that form and this in turn affects the amount of oxygen your cells receive. When you do high level thinking you need a lot of oxygen.

CHAPTER 10: SICKNESSES FROM EXCESS PHOSPHORUS

Hyperphosphatemia

Hyperphosphatemia occurs when your serum phosphorus level exceeds 2.6mEq/L and when your kidneys cannot excrete your excess phosphorous or when damage cells spill out excess phosphorous. An increase in dietary phosphorous can also cause Hyperphosphatemia. And, if you overuse laxatives that contain phosphates or do phosphate enemas, you will have an increase of phosphorous in your body.

Sodas

Sodas have a high quantity of phosphorus. The danger of drinking a lot of sodas is that your phosphorus levels will increase and this will affect the level of body calcium. Phosphorus and calcium balance each other in your body and work together to build bones. Excess phosphorus decreases your calcium levels by binding or combining with it.

In this case, to decrease your phosphorus levels, you need to decrease your soda intake to one a day or none at all.

Another issue is that phosphorus also binds with magnesium, manganese, zinc and copper, which infers with the work these minerals need to do.

So, don't drink regular, caffeine-free, diet, and club sodas.

Protein

When you eat meat, you lose calcium. Since meat is acidic, calcium is used to neutralize this acid and in doing so affects the balance of phosphorus. If you don't have enough calcium in your body stores, calcium will be pulled from your bones.

Meat protein is more acidic than the protein in fish, nuts, seeds, beans, and dairy products so less calcium is lost when you eat these foods.

The kidneys are responsible for most of the phosphorous excretion. They usually excrete the same amount that is absorbed through the digestive system. But, when they don't, your body has more phosphorous than it needs. When the thyroid or parathyroid is damage or malfunctions, PTH hormone, which regulates phosphorous excretion from the kidney, is decreased causing an increase phosphorous in your body.

Transcellular shift of phosphorous in cells, movement of phosphorus in and out of your cells, can cause a rise in body phosphorous levels. Here is a list of problems that can cause transcellular shifts.

Acid-base imbalances
Cellular destruction
Chemotherapy
Muscle necrosis
Infections
Heat stroke
Trauma

An excess intake of phosphorous also increases body phosphorous. This increase can come from excess use of phosphorous or vitamin D supplements, laxatives, and enemas.

One problem that can cause Hyperphosphatemia is a decrease in calcium or hypocalcemia, since these minerals have an inverse relationship, an increase in one follows a decrease in the other. This results in bone weakness or osteoporosis. In acute Hyperphosphatemia, the symptoms are usually caused by hypocalcemia, loss of calcium.

Here are a few symptoms of **Hyperphosphatemia**:

Osteoporosis

Seeks out psychics-palm readers, wants to know about his future
Feels he is superior and more knowledgeable
Excessive expression or happy emotions
Over works his mind
Detest daily routine matters
Tends toward occult subjects, spiritual and mystical activities

Chapter 11: Phosphorus Foods For Your Brain

When you lack phosphorous in your body the best way to correct this is through diet, eating high phosphorous foods, and through supplementation. The body always knows how much phosphorus and other minerals it needs. So any excess it will excrete, if your body is working well.

The highest foods in phosphorous, for your brain, are:

Meat, egg yolk, fish, dairy products, Cottage cheese, Beef Liver, dried fruits

The highest foods in phosphorous for bone building are:

Almonds, rice bran, wheat bran, pumpkin, squash, seeds, lentils, soybeans, sunflower seeds

Here is an additional list of high phosphorous foods:

Almonds, barley, bass, lentils, Beans, milk, millet, oats, Fish, bone broth, cabbage, olives, Cardamom, pecans, carrots, cashews, Cheese, rice bran, rye, sardines, Cod roe, corn, Dulse, sole, Trout, real butter, halibut, haddock, Artichoke

Meat

Meat contains 22 times more phosphorus than calcium, so this creates a nutritional imbalance, since your body needs both these minerals in same amounts. When you have an excess of phosphorus, it will deplete that calcium in your body. The reason is that calcium is needed to digest phosphorus.

When you are not low in phosphorus, it is best not to load up on meat. Eating too much meat can cause deficiencies in vitamin B6, vitamin B3, and magnesium. In addition, your body produces ammonia after metabolizing meat. It has been found that ammonia is a dangerous carcinogen and one of the causes of colon cancer. So for a good diet, eat small amounts of meat and eat plenty of nuts, fruits, and vegetables.

Nuts

One of the overall great foods to eat is nuts and almonds. They should be at the top of your list for phosphorus. The phosphorus they contain in 2/3 cup is 475mg.

Cottage cheese

Cottage cheese has around 150 mg. of calcium per cup and is low in fat. Many nutritionists feel that a high fat content can decrease your absorption of calcium. In addition, cottage cheese has a good ratio of calcium to phosphorus that makes this food a great balanced mineral food.

Beef liver

Beef liver is also very high in phosphorus. Eating 3 1/2 oz. of beef liver gives you 476 mg of phosphorus. Eat only organic liver or range liver, since other types of liver may have too many toxins.

Sodas

Sodas are so popular that many people can't eat their meal without them. Sodas do not have any health benefits and the energy boost you get from them comes from sugar and caffeine that they have.

Because sodas have high phosphorus content, they may interfere with your calcium absorption. Their sugar and phosphoric acid that they contain can lead to weight gain and tooth decay. Read the soda label, so that you know what you are drinking. Most colas and pepper flavored sodas contain large amount of phosphorus. For children this could result in restlessness or sleepiness. Children should not drink sodas and adults should use them sparingly.

CHAPTER 12: PHOSPHORUS SUPPLEMENTS

Typically, you don't need to take a supplement for phosphorus, since foods can supply plenty of it. But if you find that you need to supplement with phosphorus, here is some information to consider.

When you take mineral supplements, you want them to be "chelated." What this means is that the mineral in question is chemically bonded to an amino acid. In the food you eat, minerals always combine with an amino acid. Your body recognizes chelated minerals and absorbs them quickly and easily. This is why fresh juices are so good because they contain minerals in chelated form.

When you have severe hypophosphatemia you will require an I.V. infusion of potassium phosphate. This is the fastest way to get phosphorus into your body.

Young adults aged 11 to 24 should have 1200 mg. of phosphorus daily. Children from 1 to 10 years require 800 mg. daily. Typically, you would get this phosphorus from the food you eat.

The adult daily recommendation for phosphorous is 800 to 1200 mg., which is easily absorbed through the Jejunum. The Jejunum is part of the small intestine and the part that follows the duodenum. The small intestine consists of the duodenum, jejunum, and ileum. The duodenum is the part that is attached to the stomach. When the stomach content is processed, it moves into the duodenum where the majority of this food is absorbed. The jejunum is the center of the small intestine and the ileum is the last part, which is attached to the large intestine or ascending colon.

Homeopathic Medicine

Neutra-Phos or Neutra-PhosX - Each tablet contains 852 mg. dibasic sodium phosphate anhydrous, 155 mg. monobasic potassium phosphate, and 130 mg. monobasic sodium phosphate monohydrate. Each tablet yields approximately 250 mg. of phosphorus, 298 mg. of sodium (13.0 mEq) and 45 mg. of potassium (1.1 mEq). This product can be purchased on the internet. You should consult with your doctor before taking this supplement.

Natrum Phos.6x – is a homeopathic supplement and can be purchased at most health food stores.

Lecithin

You can buy lecithin in granule form or in capsules. It is best to take it in granule form and add it to your salads, soups, cereal, or other food you like. You can use a tablespoon each time you use it. It has little taste and it is soft. Keep it in your refrigerator to keep it fresh.

Phosphorous is a creator of light in the body and promotes intellect, thinking, higher reasoning, and abstract thoughts. It is a brain nutrient and is brought into the brain by lecithin, which is found in meat, egg yolk and fish. It improves nerve function and brain nutrition.

It is also active in creating bone matrix and this phosphorous comes from fruits and vegetables. It affects muscle tissue and is necessary for sexual function and reproduction.

In deficiency, phosphorous creates body weakness, brain fatigue and slow thinking, sensitivity to noise and criticism, lack of confidence, and lack of oxygen.

In excess, phosphorous creates optimism and idealism, volatile emotions, tissue breakdown, over confidence, and a highly vivid imagination.

Bone Meal

Bone meal is a good source of phosphorus and comes in tablets or powder. Look for bone meal that is raw, unheated, and from South America.

Use the number of tablets per day listed on the bottle or 1/2 tablespoon.

About The Author And Resources

Get one of my best kindle books *free* by going here:

http://natural-remedies-thatwork.com/optin.html

Rudy Silva is a natural consultant nutritionist educated in the United State in Nutrition and Physics. He is a graduate from the San Jose State University in California. He is author of 30 other e-books on natural remedies. He has authored a newsletter in natural remedies for over 4 years. He has many websites promoting special recommended products and information.

Resource page

Here are some of the other kindle e-books and paperback books about natural remedies that have been written by this author. You can see the entire list at:

http://tinyurl.com/b2f7wd3

Acne Remedies
Best natural acne treatments: Acne facial

Constipation Remedies
Best Constipated Women Natural Cures
How to Relieve Constipation with Fruits
Natural Constipation Remedies: Get These Natural Remedies to Eliminate Constipation

Essential Fatty Acids
Taking The Mystery out Of Essential Fatty acids

Amazing Fish Oil Benefits Revealed

Nutrition Remedies
Updated Version - Secret Diet and Nutrition
Secret Healthy Fruit Practices Revealed
Fast Healing Juice Nutrition Therapy: Nutrition Tips 3
Fantastic Alkaline Fruit Benefits Revealed
Calcium (Discover How To Use Calcium to Avoid Devastating Diseases)
Magnesium Nutrition Revealed
Best Nutrition Health Practices
Potassium Health Secrets Revealed
Phosphorus, the Best Brain Food
A Sodium Diet (What You Must Know About Sodium)
Vegetables and Vegetable Juice Cures

Stomach Remedies
Acid Reflux: Fast and Easy Cures for Acid Reflux
Asthma Treatment Cures With Remedies
How to Do Natural Colon Cleansing
Gastrointestinal Digestion Secrets Revealed

Misc. Remedies
Natural Hair Loss Treatment: Women and Men
Effective Natural Hemorrhoids Treatment
Iron Deficiency Anemia
Secrets to Understanding Behavior
Fast Acting Ear Infection Remedies
Best Impotence Health Diet
What Is a Hiatus Hernia?
Best Varicose Vein Treatments?

Men's Health
Best Impotence Health Diet

Weight loss
Ten (10) Day Quick Success Weight Loss Program: A new approach to losing weight by changing your eating habits for life

To see all of the kindle books written by this author, go to this the Authors Profile Page or this URL:

http://tinyurl.com/b2f7wd3

If you need support or want to promote any of his e-books, please contact him at rss41@yahoo.com and expect a reply within 24 hours. He looks forward to hearing from you and is happy to help you understand his material on natural and nutritional health.

Give a Review

And, don't forget to give a review for this book at Amazon.

It's not hard to give a review. It can be only a sentence or two. You don't have to leave a long review. A short review helps other people decide if they want to buy a book. So give a short review and give your thoughts to help other people and to help the author improve his book.

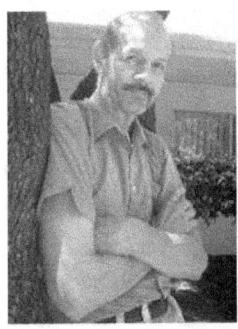

To you, for creating better health and more happiness in your life,

Rudy S Silva